# HERBS FOR HYPERTENSION

## A Natural Approach to Lowering Blood Pressure

## Dr Philip Ortner

# Table of Contents

# CHAPTER 1

## Introduction

High blood pressure, or hypertension, is a condition that affects millions of people around the world. While it might not always show obvious symptoms, its impact on our health can be profound. In this chapter, we will delve into the basics of what high blood pressure is, why it matters, and the conventional methods used to manage it. We'll also introduce the exciting realm of herbal alternatives, offering a natural approach that may complement or even replace traditional treatments.

## Definition and Significance of High Blood Pressure

Imagine your circulatory system as a well-managed network of roads and highways. Blood, the life-sustaining liquid, flows through these vessels, delivering essential nutrients and oxygen to every part of your body. Now, when the force of blood against the walls of these vessels becomes consistently too high, we enter the territory of high blood pressure.

To put it simply, blood pressure is the measure of the force of blood pushing against the walls of the arteries. The two values you often hear – systolic and diastolic – represent the pressure during the heartbeat and the pressure when the heart is at rest, respectively. Normal blood pressure keeps this force within healthy limits, ensuring that our vital organs receive the right amount of blood without straining the circulatory system.

However, when this pressure rises persistently, it can damage arteries, the heart, and other organs. Think of it as a garden hose – when water flows at an appropriate pressure, it irrigates the plants effectively. But turn up the pressure too high, and the hose may burst. Similarly, high blood pressure puts a strain on our blood vessels, increasing the risk of serious health issues such as heart disease, stroke, and kidney problems.

## Overview of the Impact on Health

High blood pressure is often referred to as the "silent killer" because it usually doesn't come with noticeable symptoms. You might feel perfectly fine, but behind the scenes, the elevated pressure can be wreaking havoc on your arteries, heart, and other organs. It's like a stealthy intruder, gradually damaging the delicate balance of your body.

One of the major concerns is its impact on the cardiovascular system. The heart, tasked with pumping blood throughout the body, has to work harder against increased resistance. Over time, this extra effort can lead to a variety of issues, including an enlarged heart, weakened heart muscles, and an increased risk of heart attacks.

The arteries, the highways of the circulatory system, face wear and tear as well. Persistent high pressure can damage the inner lining of arteries, promoting the accumulation of cholesterol and other substances, forming plaques that narrow the vessels. This process, known as atherosclerosis, further raises the risk of heart disease and stroke.

But it's not just about the heart and arteries. High blood pressure can also impact the kidneys, leading to kidney disease or failure. Additionally, it can affect the eyes, potentially causing vision problems or even blindness. The nervous system isn't spared either, as hypertension is linked to cognitive decline and an increased risk of dementia.

## Brief Discussion of Conventional Treatments and Their Limitations

Now, when it comes to managing high blood pressure, conventional medicine has its arsenal of weapons. Medications, such as diuretics, beta-blockers, and ACE inhibitors, are commonly prescribed to regulate blood pressure. These drugs work by either reducing the volume of blood or relaxing and widening the blood vessels, easing the strain on the heart.

While these medications can be effective, they are not without their drawbacks. Side effects, ranging from dizziness to fatigue, can impact the quality of life. Moreover, they often need to be taken continuously, which can be a lifelong commitment. For some, the idea of relying on pharmaceuticals for an extended period raises concerns about potential long-term effects and dependency.

Lifestyle changes, such as adopting a heart-healthy diet, regular exercise, and stress management, are also part of the conventional approach. However, these changes can be challenging to implement consistently, and their effectiveness varies from person to person.

## Introduction to the Use of Herbs as an Alternative Approach

This is where the world of herbs steps in. Imagine having a garden filled with nature's pharmacy – plants that, when used wisely, may offer a gentler yet effective way to manage high blood pressure. Herbs have been part of human healing traditions for centuries, and their potential benefits are increasingly recognized by both traditional wisdom and modern science.

In this book, we'll explore a variety of herbs that have shown promise in supporting blood pressure management. These natural remedies, when combined with lifestyle adjustments, offer a holistic approach that considers the interconnectedness of our body systems. The goal is not just to lower blood pressure but to promote overall well-being.

It's important to note that herbs are not a magical cure-all. They are tools that, when used thoughtfully, can contribute to a healthier life. Before embarking on this herbal journey, it's crucial to consult with healthcare professionals, especially if you're already on medication. The combination of herbs and conventional treatments requires careful consideration to ensure safety and effectiveness.

So, welcome to the exploration of herbs for hypertension – a journey into the world of natural remedies that, when combined with knowledge, intention, and a commitment to your health, may offer a path towards balanced blood pressure and a more vibrant life.

# CHAPTER 2

## Understanding High Blood Pressure

High blood pressure, or hypertension, isn't a condition that emerges out of nowhere. It's often the result of a combination of factors, many of which are influenced by our lifestyle choices. In this chapter, we'll dive into the factors that contribute to hypertension, explore how our daily decisions affect blood pressure, and highlight the crucial role of dietary habits and stress management in maintaining a healthy cardiovascular system.

## Explanation of the Factors Contributing to Hypertension

To understand high blood pressure, it's helpful to picture your circulatory system as a finely tuned machine. Imagine your heart as a powerful pump and your arteries as the interconnected highways that transport blood to every nook and cranny of your body. Now, let's explore what happens when things go awry.

One major factor contributing to hypertension is the narrowing of the arteries. Think of these arteries as the roads in your circulatory system, and blood as the traffic moving through them. When these roads become too narrow due to factors like plaque buildup (a combination of cholesterol, fat, and other substances), it's like trying to funnel rush-hour traffic through a single lane. The result is an increase in pressure.

Another contributor is an increased volume of blood. Imagine your circulatory system as a plumbing system. If there's more water flowing through the pipes than they can handle, the pressure in the system goes up. Similarly, if your body retains too much fluid or produces more blood than necessary, it can lead to elevated blood pressure.

The force of the heartbeat also plays a role. Each time your heart beats, it's pushing blood into the arteries. If the heart has to work harder to pump this blood, the pressure in the arteries goes up. Conditions like an overactive thyroid or certain heart problems can contribute to this increased force.

Additionally, the elasticity of the arteries matters. Healthy, flexible arteries can expand and contract as needed. However, when they become stiff and less flexible, the pressure can rise. This stiffening can result from aging, but lifestyle factors like smoking and a diet high in salt can accelerate this process.

Finally, genetics can't be ignored. Just as some families may share a tendency toward certain physical traits, they can also share a predisposition to high blood pressure. This doesn't mean genetics determine your destiny, but it highlights the importance of being vigilant if hypertension runs in your family.

Understanding these factors provides a foundation for tackling high blood pressure. It's not just about the numbers on the blood pressure cuff; it's about addressing the underlying issues that contribute to those numbers.

## Discussion on Lifestyle Choices Affecting Blood Pressure

Our daily choices play a significant role in the development and management of high blood pressure. It's like steering that finely tuned machine – the circulatory system – towards health or towards the risk of hypertension.

**Physical Activity:** Imagine your body as a car engine. Regular physical activity is like giving that engine a chance to rev up and burn off excess energy. When we engage in activities like brisk walking, swimming, or cycling, our heart gets a workout, becoming more efficient in pumping blood. This, in turn, helps to regulate blood pressure. On the flip side, a sedentary lifestyle is like letting the engine idle for too long – it becomes sluggish, and the risk of high blood pressure increases.

**Tobacco and Alcohol Use:** Smoking and excessive alcohol intake are akin to pouring sludge into the engine oil of our circulatory system. Both can contribute to the narrowing of arteries, making it harder for blood to flow smoothly. Smoking, in particular, introduces harmful chemicals into the bloodstream, accelerating the process of artery damage and plaque formation.

**Weight Management:** Picture your body weight as the cargo in the car of your circulatory system. When there's too much cargo, the engine has to work harder, and the pressure in the system goes up. Maintaining a healthy weight is like optimizing the cargo – it ensures the engine functions smoothly, reducing the strain on the heart and arteries.

## Importance of Dietary Habits

Now, let's open the hood and explore the fuel that powers our circulatory engine: our diet. Just as a car needs high-quality fuel to run efficiently, our bodies need the right nutrients to maintain a healthy cardiovascular system.

**Sodium Intake:** Imagine sodium as the salt you sprinkle on your food. While we need some salt for various bodily functions, too much can lead to water retention and an increase in blood volume. This, in turn, raises blood pressure. It's like adding too much salt to a recipe – the dish becomes unpalatable. Similarly, an excess of sodium can make your circulatory system less palatable to your overall health.

**Potassium-Rich Foods:** On the flip side, potassium-rich foods are like the secret ingredient that enhances the flavor of the dish. Potassium helps balance sodium in the body, promoting healthy blood pressure. Foods like bananas, oranges, spinach, and potatoes are rich in potassium and contribute to a well-rounded, heart-healthy diet.

**Whole Grains and Fiber:** Imagine whole grains and fiber as the slow-burning fuel for your circulatory engine. Foods like whole wheat, oats, fruits, and vegetables provide a steady release of energy, helping to maintain stable blood sugar levels and support overall cardiovascular health.

## Stress Management

Now, let's talk about stress – the traffic jam on the road to good health. In our modern lives, stress is like encountering a series of red lights during rush hour. When stress becomes chronic, it can contribute to high blood pressure in several ways.

**Hormonal Impact:** Imagine stress hormones as traffic police directing the flow of vehicles. When stress hormones like cortisol are constantly elevated, it's like having those traffic police working overtime, creating chaos in the system. This hormonal imbalance can contribute to increased heart rate and narrowed arteries, elevating blood pressure.

**Unhealthy Coping Mechanisms:** Just as some people might cope with traffic jams by honking and getting frustrated, others cope with stress in unhealthy ways.

Emotional eating, smoking, or excessive alcohol consumption are like detours that lead to a dead-end. These coping mechanisms might provide temporary relief, but in the long run, they contribute to the development and exacerbation of high blood pressure.

**Mind-Body Connection:** Consider stress management techniques like meditation, deep breathing, and yoga as the traffic signals that keep the flow moving smoothly. These practices engage the parasympathetic nervous system, promoting relaxation and counteracting the effects of stress hormones.

In summary, understanding high blood pressure involves recognizing the interplay of various factors, many of which are influenced by our daily choices. It's about navigating the roads of our circulatory system with care, making choices that promote a smooth and efficient journey towards cardiovascular health.

As we continue our journey through this book, we'll explore how herbs can be allies in this adventure, offering support in conjunction with lifestyle changes. Together, we'll build a roadmap to healthier blood pressure and a more vibrant life.

# CHAPTER 3

## Herbal Foundations for Blood Pressure Management

Welcome to the heart of our journey – the exploration of herbs as allies in the quest for balanced blood pressure. In this chapter, we'll step into the rich world of herbal remedies, introducing key plants renowned for their blood pressure-regulating properties. As we navigate this herbal terrain, we'll also take a glance at the scientific studies that lend credibility to these ancient healers. Finally, we'll explore how herbs can seamlessly complement lifestyle changes, creating a holistic approach to blood pressure management.

## Introduction to Key Herbs Known for Their Blood Pressure-Regulating Properties

Imagine a garden where each plant has a unique role in maintaining balance – this is the essence of herbal remedies for blood pressure management. These plants aren't just random foliage; they are time-tested contributors to cardiovascular health.

1. **Hawthorn (Crataegus):** Picture hawthorn as a gentle guardian of the heart. This herb has a long history of use in traditional medicine for cardiovascular issues. It is believed to dilate blood vessels, improving blood flow and reducing the workload on the heart. Think of it as widening the roads in our circulatory system, allowing traffic to flow smoothly.

2. **Garlic (Allium sativum):** Envision garlic as a culinary hero with hidden medicinal powers. Beyond its ability to add flavor to dishes, garlic has been associated with blood pressure reduction. It's like the superhero that fights against the forces narrowing our arterial roads, promoting relaxation and widening.

3. **Olive Leaf (Olea europaea):** Think of olive leaf as a peacekeeper in the circulatory system. This

herb is believed to relax blood vessels and reduce inflammation, contributing to lower blood pressure. It's like a diplomat negotiating with the traffic police to ease the flow.

4. **Hibiscus (Hibiscus sabdariffa):** Imagine hibiscus as a vibrant bloom that brings beauty and health. This herb is known for its diuretic properties, helping the body eliminate excess fluid. It's like opening a drainage system in our circulatory roads, preventing congestion and reducing pressure.

5. **Turmeric (Curcuma longa):** Visualize turmeric as a golden shield protecting the heart. This spice, with its active compound curcumin, is recognized for its anti-inflammatory and antioxidant properties. It's like adding a layer of protection to our circulatory system, reducing the risk of damage.

6. **Bilberry (Vaccinium myrtillus):** Picture bilberry as a tiny but potent ally. This herb is rich in antioxidants and is believed to strengthen blood vessels, promoting better elasticity. It's like

reinforcing the walls of our arterial roads, making them more resilient to pressure.

7. **Oregano (Origanum vulgare):** Imagine oregano as a flavorful defender against hypertension. This herb is not just for spicing up your pizza; it contains compounds that may contribute to lowering blood pressure. It's like a culinary warrior fighting against the factors that elevate pressure.

These herbs, when used judiciously and as part of a holistic approach, can be powerful allies in the quest for balanced blood pressure. However, it's important to approach herbal remedies with respect and knowledge. Always consult with healthcare professionals, especially if you are on medication or have pre-existing health conditions.

## Overview of Scientific Studies Supporting Herbal Interventions

Now, let's put on our detective hats and explore the evidence behind these herbal claims. Scientific studies provide a critical lens, helping us separate anecdote from efficacy.

1. **Hawthorn:** Numerous studies have explored the cardiovascular benefits of hawthorn. Research suggests that hawthorn may improve symptoms of heart failure, enhance exercise tolerance, and contribute to a modest reduction in blood pressure. It's like having a scientific stamp of approval on hawthorn's role in cardiovascular health.

2. **Garlic:** Garlic has been a subject of scientific curiosity for decades. Studies have indicated that garlic may have a modest effect on blood pressure, particularly in individuals with hypertension. It's like the scientific community acknowledging garlic's potential as more than just a kitchen staple.

3. **Olive Leaf:** Research on olive leaf extract suggests potential benefits for blood pressure management. Olive leaf's antioxidant and anti-inflammatory properties may contribute to its

cardiovascular effects. It's like uncovering the scientific rationale behind this ancient remedy.

4. **Hibiscus:** The vibrant hibiscus has caught the attention of researchers, and studies indicate its potential to lower blood pressure. Hibiscus tea, in particular, has been associated with a decrease in both systolic and diastolic blood pressure. It's like science recognizing the health benefits hidden in a cup of herbal tea.

5. **Turmeric:** Curcumin, the active compound in turmeric, has been extensively studied for its anti-inflammatory properties. While more research is needed, some studies suggest a potential role in blood pressure regulation. It's like uncovering the golden potential of turmeric beyond its culinary charm.

6. **Bilberry:** Scientific interest in bilberry has grown, with studies exploring its antioxidant and vascular protective effects. While more research is needed to establish a direct link to blood pressure, the preliminary findings are promising. It's like

shining a scientific spotlight on this small but mighty herb.

7. **Oregano:** Oregano's potential cardiovascular benefits are still an emerging area of study. Some research suggests that oregano may have anti-hypertensive effects, but more investigation is required. It's like starting to unravel the mysteries of oregano beyond its role in the kitchen.

While these studies provide valuable insights, it's crucial to approach them with a discerning eye. Scientific research is an ongoing process, and the field of herbal medicine continues to evolve. Always consult with healthcare professionals and consider the broader context of your health when incorporating herbs into your routine.

## How Herbs Complement Lifestyle Changes for Holistic Management

Imagine lifestyle changes as the steering wheel, guiding our journey towards balanced blood pressure. Now, picture herbs as the navigational tools that fine-tune our path, enhancing the overall effectiveness of these changes.

1. **Dietary Harmony:** Herbs can be culinary companions, enriching our meals with flavor and health benefits. Integrating herbs like garlic, turmeric, and oregano into our diet is like adding natural seasoning to our cardiovascular health. They complement the efforts of a heart-healthy diet, contributing not only to taste but also to the overall well-being of our circulatory system.

2. **Stress Reduction:** Herbs, through their calming and adaptogenic properties, can be allies in stress management. Incorporating practices like sipping hibiscus tea or using adaptogenic herbs like holy basil is like adding an extra layer of tranquility to our stress-reduction journey. They synergize with mindfulness techniques, helping to keep stress hormones in check and promoting relaxation.

3. **Physical Activity Support:** Some herbs, with their potential to improve blood flow and cardiovascular function, can be companions on the road to physical activity. Picture hawthorn as a gentle supporter, enhancing the benefits of exercise by promoting healthy blood circulation. It's like having a herbal workout partner that aligns with your commitment to an active lifestyle.

4. **Weight Management Assistance:** Certain herbs, by promoting metabolism and aiding digestion, can play a supportive role in weight management. Visualize herbs like turmeric and oregano as helpers in the kitchen, contributing not only to taste but also to the body's ability to process nutrients efficiently. They align with your efforts to maintain a healthy weight, creating a holistic approach to cardiovascular health.

5. **Overall Well-Being:** Herbs, with their antioxidant and anti-inflammatory properties, contribute to the overall well-being of the body. Picture them as guardians, standing watch over the health of your

arteries and heart. They complement lifestyle changes by addressing underlying factors that contribute to high blood pressure, fostering a holistic and sustainable approach.

# CHAPTER 4

## Herbs in the Kitchen

Welcome to the heart of your home, the kitchen, where the alchemy of flavors meets the science of health. In this chapter, we'll explore the delightful integration of blood pressure-friendly herbs into your daily meals. From simple cooking tips to delicious recipes, we'll journey through the culinary landscape, discovering how these herbs not only elevate the taste of your dishes but also contribute to the management of hypertension. Let's turn your kitchen into a healing haven.

## Incorporating Blood Pressure-Friendly Herbs into Daily Meals

Imagine your spice rack as a treasure trove of health, where each herb holds the potential to transform your meals into heart-healthy delights. Here's how you can seamlessly incorporate blood pressure-friendly herbs into your daily culinary repertoire:

1. **Garlic:** This aromatic gem isn't just for warding off vampires; it's a powerhouse for cardiovascular health. Start your day by sautéing minced garlic in olive oil for a heart-healthy base for your scrambled eggs. Roast vegetables with garlic for a flavorful side dish, or add it to your favorite soups and stews.

2. **Basil:** Fresh basil is like a fragrant burst of summer in your kitchen. Create a simple caprese salad with tomatoes, mozzarella, and basil drizzled with balsamic glaze. Toss basil into your pasta dishes or blend it into a pesto for a versatile sauce that pairs well with whole-grain pasta or grilled chicken.

3. **Oregano:** A staple in many kitchens, oregano is more than just a pizza topping. Sprinkle dried oregano onto roasted vegetables or add it to your tomato-based sauces for a robust flavor. Marinate chicken or fish with olive oil, lemon, and oregano for a heart-healthy and tasty dish.

4. **Turmeric:** This golden spice can add both color and health benefits to your meals. Create a turmeric-infused rice by adding a pinch of turmeric to your cooking water. Blend turmeric into smoothies or soups, or create a golden latte with turmeric, ginger, and a splash of almond milk.

5. **Rosemary:** The fragrant and woody aroma of rosemary can elevate various dishes. Roast potatoes with olive oil and chopped rosemary for a delightful side dish. Infuse olive oil with rosemary to drizzle over salads or use it as a marinade for grilled vegetables or meats.

6. **Thyme:** With its subtle earthy flavor, thyme is a versatile herb for both savory and sweet dishes. Add fresh thyme to roasted carrots or sweet potatoes. Mix thyme into a honey-lemon glaze for a delicious topping for grilled chicken or fish.

7. **Cilantro:** This bright and citrusy herb is a staple in many cuisines. Create a refreshing salsa with tomatoes, onions, and cilantro to accompany grilled fish or chicken. Sprinkle cilantro over

salads, tacos, or stir it into your favorite curry for a burst of fresh flavor.

## Recipe Ideas and Cooking Tips for Hypertension Management

Now that we've invited these herbs into our kitchen, let's explore some simple yet delectable recipes and cooking tips designed with hypertension management in mind:

1. **Heart-Healthy Stir-Fry:**
   - Ingredients: Mixed vegetables (broccoli, bell peppers, snap peas), lean protein (chicken, tofu), garlic, ginger, low-sodium soy sauce, sesame oil.
   - Cooking Tip: Sauté garlic and ginger in sesame oil for a flavorful base. Add vegetables and protein, stir-frying until just tender. Finish with a drizzle of low-sodium soy sauce.
2. **Mediterranean Quinoa Salad:**

o Ingredients: Cooked quinoa, cherry tomatoes, cucumber, feta cheese, olives, basil, olive oil, lemon juice.

o Cooking Tip: Mix fresh basil into the salad for a burst of flavor. Dress with a simple vinaigrette made with olive oil and lemon juice. Add grilled chicken for a protein boost.

3. **Turmeric-Ginger Smoothie:**

o Ingredients: Banana, frozen mango, yogurt, almond milk, turmeric, ginger.

o Cooking Tip: Blend frozen mango with a ripe banana, a spoonful of yogurt, almond milk, and a pinch of turmeric and ginger. This smoothie is a tasty way to incorporate anti-inflammatory herbs into your morning routine.

4. **Garlic and Rosemary Roasted Vegetables:**

o Ingredients: Assorted vegetables (potatoes, carrots, Brussels sprouts), garlic, rosemary, olive oil.

- Cooking Tip: Toss vegetables with minced garlic, chopped rosemary, and olive oil. Roast until golden brown for a flavorful and heart-healthy side dish.

5. **Herb-Infused Water:**
   - Ingredients: Fresh herbs (mint, basil), sliced cucumber, lemon slices.
   - Cooking Tip: Create a refreshing infused water by combining fresh herbs, cucumber slices, and lemon in a pitcher. Let it chill in the fridge for a couple of hours for a hydrating and flavorful drink.

# Culinary Herbs and Their Health Benefits

Let's take a closer look at how these culinary herbs contribute not just to the taste of our dishes but also to our overall health:

1. **Garlic:** Known for its potential to lower blood pressure and cholesterol, garlic is a versatile herb

that adds depth to various dishes. Its sulfur compounds are believed to have vasodilatory effects, helping to relax blood vessels.

2. **Basil:** Beyond its aromatic appeal, basil contains compounds like eugenol, which may have anti-inflammatory and antioxidant properties. These properties contribute to overall cardiovascular health and may help in managing blood pressure.

3. **Oregano:** This herb is rich in antioxidants, including rosmarinic acid and thymol, which may have anti-inflammatory effects. Oregano's potential cardiovascular benefits make it a flavorful addition to a heart-healthy diet.

4. **Turmeric:** The active compound in turmeric, curcumin, is celebrated for its anti-inflammatory and antioxidant properties. While more research is needed, some studies suggest that turmeric may have a role in blood pressure regulation.

5. **Rosemary:** With its unique aroma, rosemary contains compounds like rosmarinic acid and carnosic acid, which may have anti-inflammatory

and antioxidant effects. These properties contribute to the herb's potential cardiovascular benefits.

6. **Thyme:** Rich in antioxidants, thyme contains compounds like thymol that may have anti-inflammatory and antimicrobial properties. While more research is needed on thyme's direct impact on blood pressure, its overall health benefits make it a valuable addition to meals.

7. **Cilantro:** This herb is not only a flavor enhancer but also a source of antioxidants. Cilantro may help in lowering oxidative stress, contributing to cardiovascular health. Including cilantro in your dishes adds a burst of freshness and potential health benefits.

Incorporating these culinary herbs into your daily meals isn't just about making your dishes more flavorful; it's about turning your kitchen into a wellness sanctuary. These herbs, with their unique flavors and potential health benefits, offer a delicious way to support your journey towards balanced blood pressure.

As you experiment with these recipes and cooking tips, remember to savor the process. Cooking with herbs isn't just about nourishing your body; it's a celebration of the senses. So, roll up your sleeves, sprinkle some basil, and let the aroma of garlic fill your kitchen – your heart will thank you for it.

# CHAPTER 5

## Herbal Teas and Infusions

Imagine a quiet afternoon, a comforting mug in hand, and the gentle aroma of herbs filling the air. In this chapter, we'll embark on a journey into the world of herbal teas and infusions, exploring not only their delightful flavors but also their potential to support blood pressure management. From preparation techniques to suggested blends, we'll discover how these soothing beverages can be both a treat for the senses and a sip towards holistic health.

## Exploration of Herbal Teas with Blood Pressure-Lowering Properties

Brewing a cup of herbal tea is like creating a potion that nourishes not only your taste buds but also your well-being. Let's explore some herbs known for their potential blood pressure-lowering properties:

1. **Hibiscus Tea:** Imagine a vibrant red cup that holds the essence of hibiscus petals. Hibiscus tea has garnered attention for its potential to reduce blood pressure. Studies suggest that compounds in hibiscus may contribute to the dilation of blood vessels, promoting a more relaxed circulatory system.

2. **Hawthorn Tea:** Picture a gentle breeze carrying the aroma of blooming hawthorn flowers. Hawthorn tea is crafted from the leaves, berries, and flowers of the hawthorn plant, traditionally used to support heart health. It is believed to enhance blood flow and promote cardiovascular well-being.

3. **Olive Leaf Tea:** Envision sipping on a warm infusion that captures the essence of olive leaves. Olive leaf tea is associated with potential blood pressure benefits. The active compounds in olive

leaves, such as oleuropein, may contribute to vasodilation, helping to ease the flow of blood through the arteries.

4. **Garlic Tea:** Think of the robust aroma of garlic in a comforting cup. While not as common as other herbal teas, garlic tea has been explored for its potential cardiovascular benefits. Garlic contains allicin, a compound that may have vasodilatory effects, supporting healthy blood flow.

5. **Green Tea:** Picture a cup filled with the freshness of green tea leaves. While it contains caffeine, green tea is rich in antioxidants called catechins. Some studies suggest that regular consumption of green tea may have a modest lowering effect on blood pressure.

## Preparation Techniques and Suggested Blends

Brewing the perfect cup of herbal tea is an art that invites you to slow down and savor the moment. Here are some preparation techniques and suggested blends to enhance your tea experience:

1. **Hibiscus and Berry Blend:**
   - Preparation: Steep dried hibiscus petals with a handful of mixed berries (such as blueberries and raspberries) in hot water for 5-7 minutes.
   - Sip and Enjoy: This vibrant blend combines the tartness of hibiscus with the sweetness of berries for a refreshing and potentially blood pressure-friendly infusion.

2. **Hawthorn and Mint Infusion:**
   - Preparation: Infuse dried hawthorn leaves and flowers with fresh mint leaves in hot water for 8-10 minutes.
   - Sip and Enjoy: The floral notes of hawthorn pair harmoniously with the invigorating freshness of mint, creating a soothing blend that may contribute to heart health.

3. **Olive Leaf and Lemon Elixir:**

- o Preparation: Steep olive leaves with a slice of fresh lemon in hot water for 6-8 minutes.

  - o Sip and Enjoy: The subtle bitterness of olive leaves is balanced by the citrusy brightness of lemon, creating a delightful elixir with potential cardiovascular benefits.

4. **Garlic and Ginger Tonic:**

  - o Preparation: Simmer minced garlic and fresh ginger in hot water for 10-15 minutes. Strain before drinking.

  - o Sip and Enjoy: This robust tonic combines the earthiness of garlic with the warmth of ginger, offering a unique and potentially heart-healthy infusion.

5. **Green Tea and Jasmine Symphony:**

  - o Preparation: Steep green tea leaves with a few jasmine flowers in hot water for 3-5 minutes.

  - o Sip and Enjoy: The delicate aroma of jasmine complements the freshness of green tea, creating a fragrant symphony that may contribute to overall well-being.

## The Role of Hydration in Hypertension Management

As we indulge in the pleasures of herbal teas and infusions, it's essential to recognize the pivotal role of hydration in the journey towards managing hypertension.

1. **Fluid Balance:** Imagine your body as a well-tuned instrument, and water as the harmonious notes that keep everything in tune. Adequate hydration helps maintain the balance of fluids in your body, supporting the optimal functioning of various systems, including your cardiovascular system.

2. **Blood Volume and Pressure:** Visualize your blood vessels as rivers that need a consistent flow to maintain balance. Hydration plays a role in regulating blood volume, influencing blood pressure. When you're well-hydrated, your blood

vessels can efficiently transport blood, contributing to a healthier circulatory system.

3. **Electrolyte Balance:** Picture electrolytes as the conductors orchestrating the symphony of bodily functions. Proper hydration helps maintain electrolyte balance, including sodium and potassium. This balance is crucial for heart health, as it influences the fluid levels in and around cells, contributing to blood pressure regulation.

4. **Stress Reduction:** Envision hydration as a soothing balm that helps manage the effects of stress. Dehydration can exacerbate stress, leading to increased levels of stress hormones. Staying adequately hydrated supports your body's ability to cope with stress, contributing to a more relaxed state.

5. **Herbal Teas as Hydration Allies:** As you enjoy herbal teas and infusions, you're not just sipping flavorful beverages; you're also contributing to your daily hydration needs. While water is the primary source of hydration, herbal teas add

variety to your fluid intake, making the process enjoyable and potentially offering additional health benefits.

# CHAPTER 6

## Herbal Supplements and Tinctures

Welcome to the realm of herbal supplements and tinctures, where the concentrated power of plants is encapsulated in convenient forms. In this chapter, we'll navigate through an overview of herbal supplements designed to support blood pressure, understand the importance of proper usage and dosage, and discuss cautionary notes on combining herbs with medications. Let's delve into the world of herbal remedies, ensuring a safe and informed journey towards balanced blood pressure.

## Overview of Herbal Supplements for Blood Pressure Support

Imagine herbal supplements as condensed potions, carefully crafted to harness the medicinal properties of plants. When it comes to blood pressure support, several herbs have taken center stage in supplement form. Here are some commonly used herbal supplements:

1. **Garlic Supplements:** Derived from garlic bulbs, these supplements often contain concentrated extracts of allicin, the active compound in garlic known for its potential blood pressure-lowering effects. Garlic supplements are popular for their cardiovascular benefits and are often used to complement dietary efforts.

2. **Hawthorn Extracts:** Harvested from the leaves, flowers, and berries of the hawthorn plant, these supplements are believed to promote heart health. Hawthorn extracts may support blood vessel dilation, leading to improved blood flow and potentially contributing to blood pressure regulation.

3. **Olive Leaf Extracts:** Extracts from olive leaves contain compounds like oleuropein, known for their antioxidant and anti-inflammatory properties. These supplements are associated with potential

cardiovascular benefits, including supporting healthy blood pressure.

4. **Fish Oil Supplements:** While not an herb, fish oil deserves a mention for its omega-3 fatty acids, particularly EPA and DHA. These fatty acids are found in abundance in fatty fish and are known for their potential to support heart health, including blood pressure management.

5. **Coenzyme Q10 (CoQ10) Supplements:** CoQ10 is a compound found in the cells of the body, and supplements are often used for various health purposes, including cardiovascular support. Some studies suggest that CoQ10 may have a modest effect on blood pressure.

6. **Turmeric/Curcumin Supplements:** Derived from the turmeric root, curcumin supplements offer a concentrated form of the active compound in turmeric. With anti-inflammatory and antioxidant properties, curcumin supplements are explored for their potential cardiovascular benefits.

## Proper Usage and Dosage Guidelines

Using herbal supplements is like adding precise ingredients to a recipe – it requires attention, understanding, and a respect for balance. Here are some general guidelines for the proper usage and dosage of herbal supplements:

1. **Consultation with Healthcare Professionals:** Before incorporating any herbal supplement into your routine, it's crucial to consult with your healthcare provider. They can provide personalized advice based on your health history, existing conditions, and medications. This step is especially important to avoid potential interactions with prescribed drugs.

2. **Start Slowly and Monitor:** When introducing a new herbal supplement, start with a lower dosage to assess your body's response. Monitor how your body reacts over time, paying attention to any changes in symptoms or side effects. Gradually

adjust the dosage based on your individual needs and tolerance.

3. **Follow Recommended Dosages:** Herbal supplements often come with recommended dosages on the product labels. These dosages are typically based on scientific research and traditional use. It's important to adhere to these guidelines and avoid exceeding recommended doses unless advised by a healthcare professional.

4. **Consider Bioavailability:** Some herbal supplements may have variations in bioavailability, which refers to the amount of the active compound that enters the bloodstream. Factors like the form of the supplement and whether it's taken with food can influence bioavailability. Discuss these considerations with your healthcare provider.

5. **Be Consistent:** Consistency is key when taking herbal supplements. Unlike pharmaceutical drugs that often require strict adherence to timing, herbal supplements are generally more forgiving.

However, establishing a consistent routine enhances their potential benefits.

6. **Understand Potential Interactions:** Certain herbs may interact with medications or other supplements. For example, garlic supplements may have anticoagulant effects, and combining them with blood-thinning medications could increase the risk of bleeding. Always inform your healthcare provider about all supplements you're taking.

7. **Quality Matters:** Choose reputable brands and products when selecting herbal supplements. The quality of the extraction process, the source of the herbs, and the overall manufacturing standards influence the effectiveness and safety of the supplement.

# Cautionary Notes on Combining Herbs with Medications

Combining herbs with medications is like orchestrating a symphony – each element needs to harmonize without discord. Here are cautionary notes to consider when combining herbs with medications:

1. **Potential Interactions:** Herbs and medications can interact in various ways. Some herbs may enhance or inhibit the effects of medications, leading to unintended consequences. For example, hawthorn may potentiate the effects of certain heart medications, requiring careful monitoring.

2. **Blood Pressure Medications:** If you're already taking prescribed blood pressure medications, adding herbal supplements that have blood pressure-lowering effects can result in an excessive drop in blood pressure. This emphasizes the importance of close collaboration with your healthcare provider.

3. **Blood-Thinning Medications:** Certain herbs, like garlic and ginkgo biloba, may have blood-thinning effects. When combined with anticoagulant medications, this can increase the risk of bleeding. It's crucial to inform your healthcare provider of all

supplements you're taking, especially if you are on blood-thinning medications.

4. **Liver Enzyme Interactions:** Some herbs may influence liver enzymes responsible for metabolizing medications. St. John's Wort, for example, is known to affect the metabolism of various drugs. Discuss any potential interactions with your healthcare provider to ensure the safe use of herbal supplements.

5. **Kidney Function:** Herbal supplements are processed by the kidneys, and certain herbs may affect kidney function. If you have kidney issues or are taking medications that impact kidney function, it's essential to discuss this with your healthcare provider.

6. **Pregnancy and Breastfeeding:** Pregnant and breastfeeding individuals should exercise caution when using herbal supplements, as the effects on the developing fetus or nursing infant may not be well understood. Consult with a healthcare

provider before incorporating herbs into your routine during these periods.

7. **Individual Sensitivities:** Just as individuals vary in their response to medications, the same holds true for herbs. Some people may be more sensitive to certain herbs or may experience allergic reactions. If you notice any adverse effects, discontinue use and consult your healthcare provider.

# CHAPTER 7

## Lifestyle Synergy

Welcome to the heart of holistic health, where the symphony of lifestyle choices harmonizes with the healing power of herbs. In this chapter, we'll dive into the essence of a holistic approach to blood pressure management. Imagine this chapter as a compass guiding you through the integration of herbal remedies with exercise, stress reduction, and sleep. Along the way, we'll weave in personal anecdotes and case studies, illuminating the transformative power of successful lifestyle changes.

## Emphasizing the Importance of a Holistic Approach

Imagine your health as a tapestry, woven from the threads of various aspects of your life. A holistic approach to blood pressure management is like tending to the entire tapestry, recognizing that each thread plays a crucial role in the overall picture. Here's why a holistic approach is paramount:

1. **Addressing Root Causes:** Blood pressure is influenced by a myriad of factors, from genetics to lifestyle choices. A holistic approach allows us to delve into the root causes rather than merely addressing symptoms. It's like looking beneath the surface of a pond to understand what creates the ripples.

2. **Creating Sustainable Change:** Holistic health is about creating lasting and sustainable change. It's not a sprint but a marathon, where each step towards balance contributes to long-term well-being. It's like planting seeds that grow into a flourishing garden of health over time.

3. **Balancing Mind and Body:** The mind-body connection is a powerful force. Stress, emotions, and mental well-being are intertwined with

physical health. A holistic approach recognizes this intricate dance, fostering balance in both mind and body. It's like tuning a musical instrument to create a harmonious melody.

4. **Maximizing Herbal Synergy:** Herbs are not standalone remedies but integral players in the holistic orchestra of health. When combined with lifestyle changes, they become synergistic elements that amplify the overall impact. It's like herbs and lifestyle choices complementing each other, creating a melody of wellness.

## Integrating Herbal Remedies with Exercise, Stress Reduction, and Sleep

Now, let's embark on the journey of integration, where herbs join hands with key lifestyle elements to orchestrate a symphony of health.

1. **Exercise as a Rhythm of Wellness:**
   - **Herbal Harmony:** Consider herbs like hawthorn and garlic as companions on your

workout journey. Hawthorn's potential to improve blood flow aligns with the increased circulation during exercise. Garlic, with its cardiovascular benefits, becomes a supportive partner in maintaining heart health.

- ○ **Practical Integration:** Engage in activities you enjoy, whether it's a brisk walk, yoga, or dancing. Infuse your routine with herbal teas, creating a hydrating and health-enhancing ritual. Picture hawthorn tea as your post-workout cooldown, supporting your heart as it returns to a resting state.

- ○ **Case Study:** Meet Sarah, who incorporated daily walks in nature and herbal teas into her routine. Over time, she experienced not just improved cardiovascular health but also a heightened sense of well-being. The rhythmic connection between herbs and movement became a cornerstone of her lifestyle.

2.  **Stress Reduction as a Melody of Tranquility:**

- o **Herbal Harmony:** Imagine herbs like chamomile and holy basil as allies in your stress reduction journey. Chamomile's calming properties and holy basil's adaptogenic effects can contribute to a more resilient response to stress.

- o **Practical Integration:** Incorporate mindfulness practices into your day, such as meditation or deep breathing exercises. Create a calming herbal infusion with chamomile and holy basil, allowing the gentle aroma and soothing warmth to envelop you in tranquility.

- o **Case Study:** Meet Alex, who introduced daily meditation and a cup of chamomile tea into his routine. The combination became a ritual that not only lowered his stress levels but also positively impacted his blood pressure. The herbal melody became a source of serenity in his daily life.

3.  **Sleep as a Lullaby for Well-Being:**

  o **Herbal Harmony:** Visualize herbs like valerian and lavender as sleep-inducing companions. Valerian's potential to promote relaxation and lavender's calming aroma can create a restful environment.

  o **Practical Integration:** Prioritize sleep hygiene by establishing a consistent bedtime routine. Brew a cup of herbal tea with valerian and lavender as part of your winding-down ritual. Picture the herbs as gentle lullabies, preparing your body and mind for a rejuvenating night's sleep.

  o **Case Study:** Meet James, who struggled with sleep disturbances. By incorporating herbal teas and adopting a bedtime routine, he experienced not only improved sleep but also a noticeable reduction in his blood pressure. The herbal lullaby became his nightly elixir of tranquility.

# Personal Anecdotes and Case Studies of Successful Lifestyle Changes:

As we journey through lifestyle synergy, let's draw inspiration from real-life stories of individuals who witnessed transformative changes through a holistic approach:

1.  **Emma's Garden of Wellness:**
    - **Background:** Emma, a 45-year-old office worker, faced high stress levels and elevated blood pressure. Inspired by the holistic approach, she transformed her balcony into a small herb garden.
    - **Integration:** Emma cultivated herbs like mint, basil, and lavender. She incorporated them into her meals, brewed teas, and used their aroma for relaxation. As her connection with nature deepened, so did her ability to manage stress, leading to improved blood pressure.

- **Outcome:** Emma's journey showcases the transformative power of nature and herbs in creating a sanctuary of well-being. Her blood pressure normalized, and she found a renewed sense of balance in her life.

2. **David's Dance of Cardiovascular Health:**
   - **Background:** David, a 50-year-old dance enthusiast, was determined to address his sedentary lifestyle and borderline hypertension.
   - **Integration:** David incorporated herbal supplements, especially garlic, into his routine to support cardiovascular health. He also joined a dance class, infusing movement into his daily life. The rhythmic dance steps became a joyful exercise, complementing the herbs' potential benefits.
   - **Outcome:** David's lifestyle synergy resulted in not just improved blood pressure but also a newfound passion for dance. The combination of herbs and movement became

his dynamic duo for cardiovascular well-being.

3. **Sophie's Symphony of Self-Care:**

   o **Background:** Sophie, a 35-year-old working mother, juggled multiple responsibilities, leading to chronic stress and erratic sleep patterns.

   o **Integration:** Sophie introduced herbal teas, incorporating chamomile and valerian into her evening routine. She also embraced mindfulness practices, such as short meditation breaks during the day. The herbs and mindfulness became notes in her symphony of self-care.

   o **Outcome:** Sophie's commitment to holistic well-being resulted in better sleep, reduced stress, and a noticeable improvement in her blood pressure. The herbal symphony became her daily ritual of self-love and rejuvenation.

# CHAPTER 8

## Navigating Your Herbal Journey

Congratulations on reaching the final chapter of your herbal journey towards balanced blood pressure. In this chapter, we'll recap the key herbs and lifestyle changes we've explored, provide guidance on creating a personalized herbal plan, share resources for ongoing support and information, and emphasize the importance of regular health check-ups and collaboration with healthcare professionals. Think of this chapter as your compass, guiding you as you navigate the path of holistic well-being.

## Recap of Key Herbs and Lifestyle Changes

Let's take a moment to reflect on the herbs and lifestyle changes that have been your companions on this journey:

1. **Hawthorn:** A herbal ally known for its potential to support heart health by improving blood flow and promoting cardiovascular well-being. Picture hawthorn as the gentle breeze that enhances the rhythm of your heart.

2. **Garlic:** A flavorful herb celebrated for its cardiovascular benefits, including potential blood pressure-lowering effects. Imagine garlic as the aromatic essence that not only adds zest to your meals but also contributes to the vitality of your arteries.

3. **Olive Leaf:** Derived from the leaves of the olive tree, this herb is associated with antioxidant and anti-inflammatory properties, potentially supporting healthy blood pressure. Visualize olive leaf as the guardian that protects and nurtures the well-being of your cardiovascular system.

4. **Herbal Teas:** From the vibrant hibiscus to the soothing chamomile, herbal teas have been your comforting companions. These infusions offer not

only delightful flavors but also potential health benefits, contributing to hydration and well-being.

5. **Exercise:** Whether it's a rhythmic walk, an invigorating dance, or a calming yoga session, movement has been your partner in promoting cardiovascular health. Picture exercise as the vibrant dance that enhances the flow of your circulatory symphony.

6. **Stress Reduction:** Mindfulness practices, deep breathing, and calming herbal infusions have formed the foundation of stress reduction. Imagine stress reduction as the tranquil space where the ripples of life find stillness, contributing to overall well-being.

7. **Quality Sleep:** Valerian, lavender, and bedtime rituals have become your allies in creating a restful haven for rejuvenation. Visualize quality sleep as the nightly lullaby that nourishes your body and mind.

# Guidance on Creating a Personalized Herbal Plan

Now that you have a palette of herbs and lifestyle choices, let's guide you in creating a personalized herbal plan that resonates with your unique needs:

1. **Reflection on Preferences:** Consider the herbs and lifestyle changes that resonate most with you. Reflect on your preferences, tastes, and daily routines. Your herbal journey should be a source of joy, so choose what aligns with your lifestyle.

2. **Start with Small Changes:** Introduce herbs and lifestyle changes gradually. Rome wasn't built in a day, and neither is a sustainable wellness plan. Start with one or two changes and allow them to become integrated into your daily life.

3. **Experiment with Combinations:** Herbs can complement each other, creating a synergistic effect. Experiment with herbal teas that combine different beneficial herbs. For example, a blend of

hibiscus and mint can offer both flavor and potential health benefits.

4. **Mindful Integration:** Be mindful of how these changes make you feel. Notice the subtle shifts in your energy, mood, and overall well-being. Your body communicates with you, so pay attention to its signals.

5. **Adapt to Seasons:** Just as nature goes through seasons, your wellness plan can adapt. Some herbs and activities may resonate more during certain times of the year. Embrace this ebb and flow, allowing your herbal journey to evolve with the changing seasons.

6. **Personalized Herbal Infusions:** Experiment with creating your herbal infusions based on your preferences. Combine herbs like chamomile, lavender, and mint for a calming bedtime blend. Let your creativity guide you in crafting herbal infusions that delight your senses.

7. **Incorporate Herbs into Meals:** Consider how you can incorporate herbs into your meals.

Experiment with garlic-infused olive oil, add fresh herbs like basil and oregano to your dishes, and explore the world of culinary herbs as both flavor enhancers and potential health allies.

## Resources for Ongoing Support and Information

As you continue your herbal journey, here are resources that can provide ongoing support and information:

1. **Herbalists and Naturopaths:** Consult with herbalists or naturopaths who specialize in holistic health. They can offer personalized guidance, taking into account your individual health needs and goals.

2. **Online Communities:** Join online communities focused on herbal remedies and holistic well-being. These platforms provide a space for sharing experiences, asking questions, and gaining insights from a community of like-minded individuals.

3. **Books and Journals:** Explore books and journals on herbalism and natural health. Authors often share in-depth knowledge, case studies, and practical tips that can deepen your understanding of herbs and their applications.

4. **Workshops and Courses:** Attend workshops or online courses on herbalism. These learning opportunities can empower you with practical skills, allowing you to confidently navigate the world of herbs and holistic health.

5. **Herb Shops and Farmers' Markets:** Visit local herb shops and farmers' markets to connect with herbalists and explore a variety of herbs. Many herbalists are passionate about sharing their knowledge and can provide guidance on selecting and using herbs.

6. **Educational Websites:** Explore reputable websites dedicated to herbal education. These sites often offer articles, guides, and resources that cover a wide range of herbal topics.

7. **Podcasts and Webinars:** Listen to podcasts and attend webinars on herbalism and natural health. These platforms feature discussions, interviews, and expert insights that can enhance your herbal knowledge.

## Encouragement for Regular Health Check-ups and Collaboration with Healthcare Professionals

While herbal remedies and lifestyle changes play a crucial role in holistic health, regular health check-ups and collaboration with healthcare professionals remain essential. Here's why:

1. **Holistic and Conventional Integration:** Holistic health and conventional medicine can work hand in hand. Your healthcare provider can provide a comprehensive understanding of your health, including factors that herbal remedies may not address.

2. **Monitoring Blood Pressure:** Regular health check-ups allow for the monitoring of your blood

pressure and overall cardiovascular health. This ensures that any changes, whether positive or concerning, are detected and addressed in a timely manner.

3. **Medication Management:** If you are on prescribed medications, collaboration with your healthcare provider is crucial. They can monitor potential interactions between herbal remedies and medications, ensuring your safety and well-being.

4. **Individualized Advice:** Healthcare professionals can offer personalized advice based on your medical history, current health status, and any existing conditions. This individualized guidance is invaluable in creating a well-rounded approach to your health.

5. **Preventive Care:** Health check-ups focus not only on addressing existing concerns but also on preventive care. Early detection of potential issues allows for proactive measures to maintain and enhance your well-being.

6. **Open Communication:** Establish open communication with your healthcare provider about your herbal journey. Share the herbs you are using, lifestyle changes you've implemented, and any observations or changes in your health. This collaboration ensures that everyone is on the same page for your well-being.

7. **Celebrating Progress:** Regular check-ups provide opportunities to celebrate your progress. Whether it's improvements in blood pressure, overall well-being, or positive lifestyle changes, your healthcare provider can offer guidance and encouragement.

In conclusion, navigating your herbal journey is a dynamic and evolving process. As you continue to explore the world of herbs and embrace holistic lifestyle changes, remember that your health is a collaborative endeavor. By combining the wisdom of herbal remedies with the expertise of healthcare professionals, you create a balanced and resilient foundation for your well-being.

May your herbal journey be a source of empowerment, vitality, and lifelong health.

www.ingramcontent.com/pod-product-compliance
Lightning Source LLC
Chambersburg PA
CBHW050746260726
48661CB00001B/448